Addictive Relationships: Why Love Goes Wrong in Recovery

Addictive Relationships: Why Love Goes Wrong in Recovery

By

Terence T. Gorski

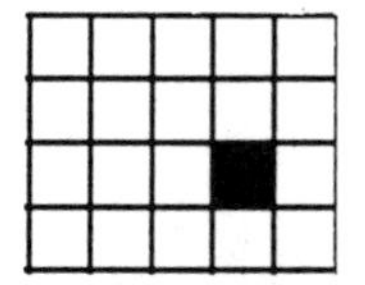

Adapted from a lecture in San Diego, California

Herald House/Independence Press
1001 West Walnut
P.O. Box 390
Independence, Missouri 64051-0390

Printed in the United States of America
ISBN 13: 9780830906369
ISBN 10: 0-8309-0636-3

Introduction

Terence T. Gorski is president of The CENAPS Corporation (The Center for Applied Sciences). CENAPS is a research, training, and consultation organization that specializes in the treatment of addictive and co-addictive disease. In his nearly twenty years of experience with the recovery process, Terry Gorski has developed a practical and no-nonsense approach to dealing with relationships in recovery.

In this presentation to 600 recovering people at an Adult Children of Alcoholics convention in San Diego, California, Terry gives four vital messages.

First, relationships are not "all or nothing" propositions. They unfold on a variety of levels, and we need to enjoy all levels of relationships.

His second message tells us to take our time building relationships. Solid love relationships aren't developed on the first date.

Third, there are addictive styles and healthy styles of relationships. If we come from a dysfunctional family, we probably don't know the difference. Until we learn what healthy relationships are all about, we will be condemned to recreate our family of origin as adults.

His final message is one of hope. There are skills and tools that can be used to build positive love relationships. We *can* recover. We *can* break the cycle of addictive intimacy.

The Functional Family

When I was invited to address this ACA group, I was asked to answer the question, "What is normal in a relationship"? In an attempt to do that, I found that I first needed answers to other questions such as, "How many people in the United States come from basically functional families"?

A functional family of origin is a family unit or home that basically equips a child with the necessary emotional, intellectual, and relationship skills to deal with life as an adolescent and as an adult. In a functional family, we learn to recognize what we feel, put labels on our feelings, and then tell other people about the feelings. Conversely, we gain the capacity to care about what others feel, to listen to their feelings, and respond to them.

A functional family also prepares children to cope intellectually with the world. It teaches them how to think clearly and accurately without major denial. It teaches them how to see reality more or less for what it is. And, finally, a healthy family teaches children how to relate in a productive manner through relationships with other human beings.

The best estimate I can give you about how many people come from healthy, functional families is somewhere around 20 to 30 percent of adults in the United States today. If you come from a dysfunctional family and happen to meet one of these people, it is a really strange experience. I found this out in a church support group. We decided to introduce ourselves by telling the stories of our childhood and I offered to go first. Afterward, I thought the four people who came from functional families were lying. I didn't believe they really got the kind of loving and caring that they said they had received. I couldn't believe they were able to identify and talk about feelings, to think clearly about reality, and to express opinions. I was amazed they had actually learned how to cope with other people.

What Is Normal?

People who come from functional families have learned unconsciously how to relate in a productive, healthy, and intimate manner with others. If you have come from a dysfunctional family, you have learned unconsciously and habitually to relate with others in a destructive style of intimacy. And, if 20 to 30 percent of the adults in the United States come from functional families, then 70 to 80 percent come from dysfunctional families.

Now if 75 percent, give or take 10 percent on either side, come from a dysfunctional family, it is "normal" in the United States today to be dysfunctional in your relationships. And if you don't believe this, I encourage you to watch television. Take a look at the role models being held up and try to recall the last successful soap opera you saw that role-modeled healthy intimate relationships. They are few and far between.

Instead of asking what is *normal* in a relationship, I'm suggesting that we ask what is *healthy* in a relationship. What does it mean to have a healthy interpersonal relationship? In this respect, I don't want to become the *norm* of this society, I want to become *abnormal*.

Communications Exercise

Healthy relationships are based on the ability to do two basic things: to identify your thoughts and feelings and to communicate them. Here's an exercise.

First, sit back, settle into your chair, take a deep breath, and notice what's going on inside the center part of your body from the pit of your stomach right up to your throat. See if you can put a word label on this feeling. Take another breath and notice if you've got a conversation going on in your head. Then, take a third deep breath and note whether your mind has a tendency to go away to someplace special.

Now come back out of yourself and turn to somebody next to you, look the person right in the eye, and say "Hello." Then share with him or her, in just a word or a phrase, what the experience of looking inside yourself was like.

The Relationship Process

This little experiment goes through the process skills necessary for having a relationship, because a relationship is simply the process of relating to another human being. In a relationship you do two things. You look within yourself to identify your inner experiences—what you are thinking, what you are feeling, and what you are imagining either through memory or projecting into the future. You pull out of yourself and connect with another human being by telling him or her the nature of that inner experience. Then, you listen to what the other person says to you in response. Those are the three basic skills of relationships.

After listening to what is going on inside your partner, you repeat the process. You listen to him or her, then you get back inside yourself and notice if your inner experience has changed. You pull yourself out, tell him or her how it's different now—what you're thinking differently, how you're feeling differently, what you're imagining differently—and then attend to what they are saying back.

It's simple only if, as a child, you have learned and have unconsciously developed the habit of doing that process over and over again. This is what healthy, functional families teach children to do from the day they are born through role modeling, practice, and correction until it becomes an unconscious habitual process. It is a process that people from dysfunctional families never learn. As a result, they, as adults, have to start the painful process of taking each one of those behaviors apart, relearning them, and doing them repeatedly until they get into the habit of doing it. Initially it's painful, but for those of you who have begun this process, it gets easier over time.

Levels, Natures, and Characteristics of Relationships

To understand the process of building a healthy relationship, we must first look at the different levels on which relationships operate. People from dysfunctional families often fail to recognize that healthy relationships can operate on a number of different levels. Problems occur when one person is operating at one level of a relationship and the other person is operating at a different level of relationship. The expectations just don't match and, all of a sudden, you're not quite getting from your partner what you think you should be getting. Your partner, though, is giving exactly what he or she chooses to give. It bends us out of shape a little bit.

The second thing we must explore is the nature of dysfunctional or addictive relationships. These are the types of relationships that alcoholics and drug dependent people tend to get into once they get sober and that adult children tend to get into once they start growing up.

Then, we're going to examine the characteristics of these relationships and compare them to their healthy counterparts. We'll see how to set up a vision or a goal of what is healthy and how we can start growing toward it. We can look at how to change our style and method of relating. And, finally, we'll look at some general steps for beginning the process of growing out of an addictive relationship style and into a healthy relationship style.

Pain or Abandonment

Most people from dysfunctional families learn early on that they have two relationship options: intense painful involvement or isolation and abandonment. "I can choose to be totally dysfunctional and intensely involved with a human being until it hurts so bad I can't stand it or I can be so completely alone that I hurt so bad I can't stand it." Life becomes a vacillation between painful loneliness and painful involvement.

Superficial Involvement

We fail to recognize that relationships operate on a continuum of levels. The first level is superficial involvement. Superficial involvement occurs in relationships when people interact in a very casual manner and have little investment in and absolutely no commitment to one another. Casual friends and short-term associates fall into this category as do waiters in a restaurant, a housekeeper in your building, or someone at work. You may say "Hello," shake hands, and never see them again, or it may be somebody in a group with whom you go out to dinner or take a raft trip down a river or a skiing trip over a weekend. These are casual relationships.

These casual relationships may be nonsexual or sexual. *Sexuality is no longer an indicator of intimacy in our culture,* and this is an important thing to recognize. Simply because someone wants to be sexual with you—whether they be male or female—does not necessarily mean they want to be intimate with you. The cultural revolution has come and gone and sexual practices have changed. People may seek only a casual, superficial involvement sexually, which is morally acceptable to many.

Most people from dysfunctional families feel guilty when they get involved in superficial relationships: "I should be so much more to him." They find themselves rescuing people from their personal problems. There's a tendency to escalate these relationships. "There's this guy I see on the elevator every day and he looks so depressed. I've just got to take him home tonight and care for him." The expectation says, "If I'm going to get involved with someone, it's going to be very intense and very committed. I have to shrink my social world to almost nothing because it's not okay to have superficial involvement." *Normal people have superficial involvements.* If a superficial friend is hurting, that's too bad but it's not your problem.

2

Companionship

The second level of a relationship is companionship. In a companionship, two people associate for the purpose of sharing common activities.

For example, I have a friend with whom I see movies. This is a shared activity. Suppose I call him up and say, "Hey, Joe, let's go see the new Charles Bronson flick."

He says, "I really don't want to do that tonight. Why don't we go do something else."

Then I say, "I really want to see the movie, thanks anyway," and I hang up the phone and call somebody else to see the movie with me. *In companionship, the activity is more important than the person* and the person becomes interchangeable. It's okay for me to want to go to a movie and to poll people until I find someone to go with me. If you say, "I really don't want to go to a movie, I want to go shopping," it's okay for me to say "no" to that companionship interaction.

Friendship

3

The next level up is the friendship level, which is a reverse of companionship. *In a friendship, two people associate for the purpose of mutual support and the enjoyment of each other.* The person is important, the activity is secondary. In friendship, I call you up and say, "I want to spend time with you," and then we decide on the context of the shared activity. If I want to see a movie and that person doesn't, we begin changing the activity because our primary goal is to spend time with each other.

People relate on many different levels at any given time. Here's an example: a husband comes home from work and he's just dying to go see a movie. His wife, who also works, is really lonely and wants to spend some good, intimate time with her husband. The husband is companion-oriented that night. He wants someone to share a movie with him. The wife is friendship-oriented that evening. She wants this person to be a friend and share an evening with her. And, if they are coming from dysfunctional families they don't recognize there are different relationship levels. They've never talked about this. So when the husband invites the wife into a companionship role by inviting her to see a movie and she rejects him by suggesting that they cuddle up on the couch in front of the television and really talk to each other, the trouble starts. The husband says, "Fine. You cuddle up in front of the television. I'm calling Jack to go see the movie." The wife gets upset, saying, "You don't love me," and an argument ensues when the real problem is that they are operating at different levels of relationship expectation.

Romantic Love

The final relationship level is romantic love. *This is a friendship in which there is shared passion, sensuality, and sexuality.* The expressed purpose of a romantic relationship is to have an intimate friend. Sexuality without a basis of friendship is not romantic love; it is a superficial relationship.

How It Works

You meet somebody superficially and you observe him or her with no commitment. You engage your brain to think, your gut to react, and you say, "Do I like this person? Do I feel good about this person? As I observe her, does she seem to be sane?" Evaluating the sanity of a prospective partner is not a terrible thing to do.

Once you decide this person is good for you, you invite him or her into a companionship. Why? Companions are interchangeable. There is limited commitment or involvement, so you are still safe.

The safest first dates are typically a movie or a dinner party with other people. The more involving or distracting the activity, where there's little opportunity for real intense alone time, the safer you are. You can also observe the other person and see how he or she interacts with others. If the person you're going out with wants to punch out the ticket taker at the movie because he had to wait in line, that might be a warning sign. If you begin to notice that this person is a little bit flaky, you bow out.

On the next level, you start treating the person as a friend by spending more unstructured time with him or her. This way, you get to know him or her as a person and you give the relationship a chance to evolve. You become a closer friend and, as the friendship develops, sexuality emerges. And I don't have this backward!

If you meet somebody and suddenly your hormones seem to take over, a different message is triggered. I hate to suggest that many of us think with that part of our body in the early part of a relationship, but it happens. If sexuality is the primary foundation of a relationship, it will lead you into a dysfunctional relationship 90 percent of the time. The relationships that survive are the ones where sexuality emerges out of the foundation of friendship and the relationship has moved through stages of superficial involvement to companionship to friendship to romantic love.

A Functional Association

It's not over once you're in love with someone. You don't die and go to heaven at that point. Your life will not be wonderful, fine, and fixed. Because then romantic love moves you into a functional association with the other person. As you begin to share your life with him or her, you make commitments to meet each other's physical, emotional, and social needs. It means if that person gets cancer, you don't walk out. You participate *together* to pay the bills, to pay the rent, to keep your house going. If you have children, you're making commitments that are not to be taken lightly. In the old days, this was called marriage. But today, it is just as often a pre-marriage arrangement called living together or cohabiting. We don't have a good word for it and we need one to legitimize it for what it is.

Functional association typically has two stages: you live together and then you get married. And when you look at it this way, normal people do not get married two weeks after they meet each other. That's not healthy. Normal people may meet someone and go to bed on the first date, but they realize half of that thrill is the aspect of danger. It's like placing one bullet in the chamber of a six-shooter and putting the gun to your head. It may be that you develop some things in common other than sexuality or perhaps you walk away with a sexually transmitted disease. It's a high-risk relationship. But, of course, when our hormones do the talking, we tend to use our sexuality to shut off the brain and emotions.

Addictive Relationships

With this in mind, let's take a look at what happens in addictive relationships. The addictive relationship moves from superficial involvement into companionship, friendship, romantic love, and functional association all in, say, about twenty-two minutes after you first meet this person.

The addictive relationship can be divided into eight characteristics. These are artificial, but they help to clarify the issue.

1. Magical or unrealistic expectations. Before you ever meet your partner, you know what this relationship is going to be. "I believe an intimate relationship is going to make my life better without the need to think better or act better. By the mere fact of my involvement with this person, every aspect of me and my life will just automatically get better and I won't have to do anything about it. I will be fixed. It will fix me or make me something I'm not with very little or no effort." *That's magical thinking.*

2. Instant gratification. Addictive relationships are based on a foundation of intense sexuality. Bells and whistles go off. You just can't wait because of tremendous animal magnetism.

If you are single and newly recovering in the ACA program, be careful when you go to a social event like a party. If you look across the room and a person leaps out at you with this huge animal magnetism, walk the other way. I don't know how this works, but when I was single in my early twenties, I consecutively dated four women who attempted suicide. Do you know how hard it is to find someone who is suicidal and to fall in love with her? And then to find four in a row? But it was easy. I was at a party and *bong!* there she was.

Instant gratification creates an immediate, intense, and continuous satisfaction. *In an addictive relationship, you expect your partner to provide you with immediate, instant, and continuous gratification anytime you want it.* Isn't that what love is all about? "I love you. Blow my mind," on demand.

Cocaine and heroine also "blow our minds" on demand. In an addictive relationship, you are looking for a living, breathing drug with the appropriate sex organs because that's what you've been taught. If you come from an alcoholic family, the only positive relationship you have ever witnessed is the love relationship between your addicted parents and their drug. As a result, even if you have chosen not to use the drug, you have witnessed that effect and its all-consuming passion. You've learned that this is the only thing that won't abandon you. You've got to get that feeling somewhere, so you select people who can provide it. And that feeling, which requires an adrenaline surge along with the sexual attraction, is typically associated with fear.

One woman who came to see me said, "I just don't understand it. I always find men who beat me."

So I said, "Well, where do you go to meet men?"

"I go to the biker bars," she answered.

I said, "Well, what do you do there?"

She said, "I put on a black leather miniskirt and I go in and find someone who I'm really attracted to. Everyone thinks these bikers are bad people, but they are really tender, caring people who are just misunderstood by society. Then, I get involved with one of these guys and he eventually beats me."

I said, "Did you ever think there might be a selection error going on here?" She looked at me quizzically. "Couldn't you try to meet men somewhere else?" I asked.

She looked at me with disgust and said, "Where do you want me to go—to church or something?"

When we began exploring this together in therapy, she discovered that when she went into these bars she was scared, and this feeling imitated the relationship of the love between her addicted parent and his chemical. She always felt fear when she witnessed this relationship. *In an addictive relationship, fear is confused with passion and excitement.* And the scary components of this are very important.

3. Dishonesty. There is a belief the relationship will be destroyed if you know everything there is to know about your partner, who also knows everything about you. "I can't be honest. He'd leave me. We wouldn't work out together. The whole thing would crumble into dust."

Then come the *no-talk* rules: "I can't talk about certain aspects of my inner experience. I can't give you feedback about your experiences and how it impacts on me." These no-talk rules are necessary to keep the fear alive, to keep the excitement alive, to keep the sexual passion going.

4. Compulsive and obsessive overcontrol. Since you can't be honest, you have to be sneaky. This starts the attempts at compulsive overcontrol. You have to keep the climate just right so the relationship will "blow your mind" on demand. You believe that without intense, continual effort, the relationship will self-destruct. There's even a belief that if you stop thinking about it, even for a minute, it will all fade away.

So you become obsessed with the relationship. You begin thinking about the relationship when it would be more appropriate to be thinking about other things. Your compulsion about the relationship becomes overwhelming.

Have you ever known a guy who meets a lady and sinks out of sight for three weeks? Everything else in his life becomes secondary. Nothing else counts. Then, the two of them briefly resurface until a friend says to him, "Hey, she's not good for you," and then he disappears again. He has totally rearranged his value system around her.

The essence of obsessive overcontrol lies in the fact that you can't talk to each other. You've got two people trying to control one another. You're both saying, "I can't tell you who I am or what I want because you'll leave me, so I'm going to trick you into giving me what I want without telling you about it." You expect the other person to read your mind, and if he or she doesn't recognize that you want something and doesn't give it to you, you get upset and try to manipulate them.

5. Lack of trust. People in addictive relationships don't trust each other. They never know what the other one is going to do. They have to trick them into being responsible. In a healthy relationship, there is rational trust.

Rational trust is the belief that the person will always act in accordance with their nature as a human being, with their natural free-flowing preferences in life. All human beings will naturally pursue what they believe to be in their best interests to the best of their ability. If you get hooked up with somebody and expect him or her to act in nonaccordance with his or her nature, it won't work.

Here's an example: I know a man who bought a cat, and he got really mad at this cat. I asked why.

"That animal walks all over everything. It climbs on bookshelves and over this and that. I've been beating that cat to keep him off the furniture and the drapes, but I can't get it to stay off my couch."

So I said, "Why are you trying to do that?"

"Because I had a dog that never went on the couch."

He expects the cat to violate its basic nature. Don't forget that important reason.

People have natures, too, and you're not going to get someone to change his or her fundamental, inherent nature. If somebody's nature doesn't fit yours, you're not going to change it. If you commit with somebody and you struggle to change their nature, it is *not* going to work.

I was in a relationship with a woman I loved very much, and we had all kinds of things in common—except one. I was work-oriented and loved living in the city. I wanted to "up" my career and needed someone to support that. She had come from out west and wanted to go back there, live in a log cabin, and work a twenty or thirty-hour per week job for just enough money to pay the rent. She wanted to spend her time listening to John Denver music on the front porch, reading books with her husband at her side, thriving on companionship, and taking hikes together in the woods.

That was her fundamental nature. Work was mine and, consequently, the relationship didn't work. It wasn't because we didn't love and care for each other; it was because one of us would have had to violate our nature to remain together.

Not every couple can build a productive relationship. Healthy people know and accept this. They go through a rational process—a screening process—saying, "Hey, will this person fit with me the way I am or will I have to change? And, if I have to change too much, I'm not interested. Aside from the normal process of growth, I'm not willing to change fundamentally who I am as a human being to accommodate anybody else. If it's not a joy to be around me the way I am, given of course that I'm not totally pathological, I am not interested in that relationship."

6. Alternating doubts. Addictive relationships encourage persistently alternating doubts about yourself and your partner. "Sometimes I think there must be something wrong with me because this relationship is failing. I must be inherently defective and feel a sense of shame, or I must be doing something wrong and feel a sense of guilt." Then you say, "It's not me, it's her," and you go into blaming and scapegoating: "There must be something inherently wrong with her."

Have you ever found yourself complaining about your partner and then find that you're talking to someone with some maturity in the program who, after an hour, says, "Gee, what is it about you that attracts someone like that? What is it about you that keeps you involved with someone like that?"

Alternating doubts all lead right back to you. If you are hooked up with the world's first-class loser, what's wrong with you that you are? Then you are led into shame and guilt. "I must be defective or I'm doing something wrong." You wallow in it until you say, "No, it's not my fault, it's her fault." You blame her but eventually you've got to come back to the issue of who made the decision to get into the relationship and who makes the decision to stay in it on a day-to-day basis. The fundamental question becomes, "Why are you in the relationship?" However, you can't ask that because you can't be honest and you have no-talk rules. And besides that, the sexual part of the relationship is so good. Wow, is it good. "Boom, we merge into one and it's a spiritual experience. We melt into the universe and our atoms become one. It's the big bang theory to the max. And other than that, I don't expect a thing from you. Just do that whenever I want you to."

7. Isolation. In addictive relationships, there's a need to protect this experience, just like the addict protects his drugs. Have you ever seen alcoholics leave their booze out so everyone can have some? Do coke addicts throw all their coke on the table and say, "Hey, help yourself!" Typically, they hide their supply. In addictive relationships, you do the same thing. You isolate. "Nobody's going to get near my partner. We're going to hole up all alone and no one is going to share in this experience we're having because nobody can understand the deep religious nature of this experience."

With the isolation, there's a need to hide the true nature of the relationship from other people. The relationship becomes a closed system. If you are an ACA, you can tell when the relationship is getting a little on the dysfunctional side because you can feel a strange feeling in the pit of your stomach when you consider bringing this partner around your ACA friends. You also have trouble inviting your ACA friends to join you in social activities because, of course, you don't want your privacy violated. Maybe it's because there is some "stinking stuff" in the relationship that you don't want to expose or look at.

8. Repeating Cycle of Pain. Finally, addictive relationships produce a repeating cycle of pain. There is a cycle of desperate action—"I'll do anything to make this relationship work"—followed by short-term intense pleasure. "My mind blows out of its circuits and it's so wonderful. It was worth the beating, it was worth the fight, it was worth the six months of ripping my guts to shreds for this one night of pleasure." And then, it blows up again. There's more pain followed by disillusionment. "Maybe this is never going to work." You blame your partner and then you start blaming yourself saying, "It is my fault; I'll try again." The cycle of desperate action repeats until you finally decide to throw away that relationship. You are at peace for a few weeks until you go to a party and see another person who starts the same process all over again.

Healthy Relationships

Healthy relationships work differently because they involve a developmental process of growing in each other's presence and progressing through levels of development.

One guy said to me, "I don't understand it. Women will go out with me the first time but they never say *yes* the second time around." I asked him to describe his typical first date.

"Well," he said, "I usually pick her up and we go to a nice, quiet restaurant where we can be all by ourselves to talk and get to know each other."

"What do you talk about?" I asked.

"I feel that I have to be rigorously honest. As soon as we sit down, I say, 'You're aware that I'm a recovering alcoholic, aren't you? Let me tell you my story.'" Then, he proceeds to repeat his entire AA story with all the incidents of past female abuse and asks, "You don't still want to go out with me, do you?"

Suppose the woman says, "It's okay that you're an alcoholic. I understand that."

"Good," he says. "I'm also a heroine addict." But, of course, this is just sharing.

Here's a rule if you want to have a healthy intimate relationship: **Don't tell your ACA story until the tenth date.**

A healthy person is going to run if a person starts telling this horrendous story of his or her life on the first date. An ACA, on the other hand, would probably marry that person.

A healthy individual says, "This smells of problems. I'm going to distance myself from this person and find someone who is able to relate in a sane, context-appropriate way for a first date." On first dates, you have to disregard the need for instant gratification. Go out, do something together, talk, have a cup of coffee, and go home. *End of first date.*

Differences of Healthy Relationships

1. Rational or realistic expectations. In contrast to the magical expectations of the addictive relationship, healthy relationships are realistic. If you are unemployed and get into a healthy relationship, the only difference is that you will then be an unemployed person with a healthy relationship. If you have a good, intimate relationship, you have a good lover, friend, and companion with whom you can talk about the stress of being unemployed. It doesn't change you or give you a job. If you are an emotionally unhappy person who has a healthy, intimate relationship, you're going to be an emotionally unhappy person with a good, intimate relationship. Nothing else is going to change except for the fact that you are now in a relationship. Marriage doesn't change things either. The only thing marriage will do is make your life worse for a little while because of the stress involved. Marriage can destroy a good love relationship because, once married, you unconsciously start acting out the wife or husband role expectations you learned in your family. It's an unconscious process that requires effort to overcome.

2. Build slowly. Where the addictive relationship demands intense personal sharing instantly, the healthy relationship builds slowly, gradually, and systematically to determine if future sharing is safe. There is a game plan. And, if you come from a dysfunctional family and start dating someone, you'd better run back to your sponsor or meeting and say, "This is what happened. Tell me what you think." You need a reality test.

When you conduct a relationship this way, it will feel abnormal because, for you, normal is addictive. I told one patient to slow down and take six to ten weeks to decide if she really wanted to get involved with this person.

"But that's almost three months," she said. "I can't wait."

"Well, how long has it been since you had a sexual relationship?" I asked.

"A year and a half, but I can't wait."

Healthy people are looking for long-term commitment, not instant gratification. The primary value of the relationship is not the shared sexual thrills. It is contentment, security, and peace of mind. Mentally healthy people plan for their best interest in the long term of their life. This, incidentally, does not go against the program. "One day at a time" doesn't mean that you don't plan. One day at a time means that you pay attention to what you're doing *now,* but you still look into the future. You don't pick a partner based solely on how he or she makes you feel today.

Building slowly frees you because you don't have to pick only perfect people to go out with on a first date. You're now selecting and walking away from anyone who triggers the gong inside of you. So who are you selecting? Boring people.

Here's another rule: **Build a self-protective mechanism into the relationship.** This is an important and vital concept, especially in early ACA recovery. Addictive relationships happen instantaneously while your hormones do the talking and thinking. There is no developmental process of getting to know each other. There is no self-protective process built into the relationship. Make sure you can protect yourself. As a matter of fact, I recommend this: **Do not go to bed on the first date.** How many dates you want to designate before sleeping together is up to you, but make a commitment to it.

Some people view sex as a casual thing. You go out on a first date, go to bed with somebody, and never hear from them again. For some this may be fine, but others find it very painful. It used to be the exclusive province of men abusing women this way, but that has changed. Women are engaging in that particular "sport" also. If you say no to sex on the first, second, or third date, you will find out if he is going to call you again. If he doesn't, he probably wouldn't have called you even if you had slept with him. So now, with this built-in self-protective mechanism, you can screen these guys ahead of time.

Here's another rule: **Never have sex with your partner if you don't genuinely feel good about him or her.** Never go to bed with somebody out of guilt or obligation. Those are the hallmarks of addictive relationships. And, above all, never go to bed with someone because you believe it will change him or her.

3. Honesty. A healthy relationship is based on rigorous honesty. Healthy people, before they make commitments interpersonally, want to share with their partner the nature of who they are. They want to know that they are accepted unconditionally and that they will not need to keep secrets. They make a commitment to be fully conscious of their partner and, as a matter of fact, they get offended when they find their partner has been keeping secrets from them—so much so that this could be grounds for ending the relationship.

Healthy relationships don't tolerate secrets. This doesn't mean that you truck out the litany of every little thing you've done in the past. You don't share every single concrete incident where you have done something wrong. You share the nature of your wrongs and past problems. You share the type of person you've been and the type of person you're becoming. And, if your partner can't handle it, there is no future there anyway. BUT... **Don't do it on the first, second, or third date.**

People going after addictive relationships are dishonest. There are things going on in their hearts and minds that they don't share with their partners because the belief is, "If I share that and they know that about me, they will not love me anymore." It's based on the belief that you are inherently unlovable.

4. Not obsessed with love. Healthy people, when they are single, are not psychotically obsessed with finding a partner. They may be obsessed with becoming a person who's worthy to be loved. If you put the same energy in becoming a person who is worthy of love, you don't have to compulsively hunt out somebody to love. Someone will find you.

When you spend all your time looking for someone else, you don't have any time to work on yourself. This was really driven home to me a few years ago when a therapist said, "Tell me about your life."

"Well, I can't find a woman worthy of love. I'm looking all the time and am dating seven or eight women right now."

"How would you describe the quality of the women you're dating?" he asked.

"Awful," I said, adding some derogatory remarks about all women.

"That's interesting," my therapist said. "I hear another reason why a high-quality woman who's interested in a caring, committed relationship would not be interested in you."

"What are you suggesting?" I asked.

"Stop getting involved with all of these women and open up space in your life so something can happen." This is how it starts. You've got to work on yourself.

Many people have looked out on the dating scene and said, "There are no quality people out there for me to get involved with." Who are you saying that about?

I've done workshops on intimacy and I've taken men on one side and women on the other and asked each, "What's your biggest problem?" The men say there are no quality women around and the women say there are no quality men. I ask if they consider themselves quality men and women, capable of love and intimacy, and they say "Yes." So I bring them together and they say, "Ick." This process is called delusional thinking. *They are basing their idea of intimate capacity on the fact that they are capable of having incredible sex with the right person.*

5. Voluntary free-flowing cooperation. A healthy person isn't very interested in a relationship that's going to take a lot of work. Healthy people expect the norm of the relationship to be voluntary, free-flowing cooperation. It's comfortable, secure, and it feels nice. You don't have to hide, struggle, walk on egg shells, control, and manipulate. Every once in a while you experience abnormal periods of problems, but you know you will solve those problems together through cooperation. Then, you will go back to the norm, which is comfort, satisfaction, and good times.

People from dysfunctional families believe the norm in a relationship is to constantly struggle and occasionally have a few moments of good feelings that they degrade back into a struggle. A lot of time and energy is spent on trying to change their partner and to fit him or her into their mold.

6. Social integration. The healthy relationship is socially integrated. When healthy people get involved in a relationship, they keep their old friends and together develop new ones as a couple. There is *my* social life, *your* social life, and *our* social life. You go outside the relationship and the family to get help, courage, and support. There are no secrets that have to be hidden from the whole world.

Addictive relationships are socially isolating and secretive. Two people meet and they disappear together for weeks. If your new partner has no friends, think about that. Weigh that into your process of getting to know that person.

7. Cycle of deepening contentment. Healthy relationships repeat a cycle of deepening contentment. There is satisfaction and contentment with a partner. When a problem develops that creates pain, it results in problem-solving behaviors. You rationally look at the problem and realize that you are not enemies. You are in this together and you put your mutual brain power together to work toward resolution. Then, your intimacy is heightened and you go back to your normal state of being content with one another.

The addictive relationship has a cycle of repeating pain that goes like this: intense pleasure, intense pain, disillusionment, blaming your partner, blaming yourself, and desperate action to make it happen all over again. Every once in a while you take a vacation from that and have a good time for a few minutes, but not too often. You're hard workers and you have to make this relationship grow. You need growth experiences.

First the Self

The possibility of healthy intimacy starts with the self. This is a fundamental principle of healthy love. You must first develop a healthy self before you develop a healthy relationship. You will only attract to you for an intimate relationship someone who approximates the level of emotional health that you have yourself. This makes it very difficult.

One man said to me, "I don't attract anyone but ugly, mean women."

So I said to him, "What is it about you that attracts ugly, mean women? What do you do to attract these people?"

I once went into personal therapy to find out why I couldn't find a suitable partner. I weighed 245 pounds and was working eighty hours a week. I did nothing but work, collapse, and sleep. I was psychotically obsessed with my work. I could not communicate and would monopolize conversations. I had underlying anger and hostility because I thought that once I got my career together, I'd automatically find a love relationship.

My therapist asked, "What kind of a woman do you want?"

"I want a young, attractive woman with a nice personality and lots of friends," I said. "She should be athletic and sports-minded, and she should have many interests and activities."

He listened to me, nodded, and then said, "Terry, I'm going to ask you a question. You may not like it. Can you handle it?"

"Yeah, sure," I said.

"What would a woman like that want with somebody like you?"

I fired that guy. There are plenty of therapists around. I didn't need that guy messing up my life.

If your elevator doesn't go all the way up most days, you're going to find that the people who are interested in an involvement with you don't really want to get to the top floor in life either. In other words, you're going to attract people at your level of development.

Healthy Principles

Healthy people know how to get out of relationships responsibly. If you have never gotten out of a relationship responsibly, I suggest that before you ever get serious about anybody, you give yourself the homework assignment of getting in and out of three relationships in quick succession. These relationships should be longer than just a weekend. None of the "Let's have a meaningful relationship...tonight" types.

It's okay to get out of a relationship that's not going to work before you commit to it and it's okay to take your time about making a commitment. But until you know you can get out of a relationship you will never be free to choose to stay in one. You will be trapped. And, when you have no choice, you will never be free to love because love is a free expression of choice. "I must love you in a free, natural, unrestrained way. If I am forcing myself because I know there is no way out, ever, and I start dreaming of you dying just so I can get out, that's not good." You can never love under those terms.

Healthy people do not lose themselves in their relationships. I am me, you are you, we are us. Catholics have a wedding ceremony that makes healthy people cringe. (Protestants have a similar version, I believe.) In it, the couple walks up to a statue of the Virgin Mary where two candles are burning. There is a third unlit candle one platform up. The groom picks up the candle that symbolizes him and the bride picks up the candle that symbolizes her; they merge their flames together to light the third candle. Then they blow out their own candles. That's not healthy.

Healthy people also recognize that when they get into a relationship, there are three categories of problems. There are my problems which I must solve on my own, hopefully with support and understanding from you, but you can't fix them. There are your problems that you've got to fix with my support and understanding. Then, there are our problems–those issues that we must work on together. At any given time in any relationship, all three categories of problems are present.

Healthy people recognize that there is no such thing as a perfect relationship. Their expectations are realistic. In a healthy relationship, two people trade one set of problems for a better set of problems. It's called progressive, developmental growth. That's what relationships are all about. You will always be struggling with problems. It is the same thing with recovery problems in the ACA program. You will never be problem free. Life is a series of problems, beginning with birth and ending with death, unless you believe in an afterlife.

Steps for Healthy Intimacy

Here are a couple of steps on how to get to healthy intimacy. Remember: First the self and *then* the possibility of healthy intimacy. If your relationships "stink," then so do you. I hate to say it that way, but we have to take a look at something here. If our relationships are really problematic, we are externalizing our beliefs about what relationships should be. Until we straighten those expectancies out, relationships will be a mirror of our inner being.

The first step is to *establish and maintain a program of personal growth and recovery.* First me, then a possibility of healthy intimacy. In your early recovery, there's nothing wrong with swearing off relationships until you get your stuff together.

Second, *establish realistic expectations of what an intimate relationship is and should be.* Establish what a relationship will and will not do for you.

Third, *select an appropriate partner.* If you are in a relationship, evaluate your partner's willingness to work with you to improve intimacy. If you are selecting a partner, you must look for these two things: That you have things in common and that you are both interested in developing the same nature of a relationship. Both of you need to be looking to develop the same level of intimacy. If one wants one level and the other wants another level, you're not going to get it together. A lot of problems in intimacy are plain and simple selection errors. ACAs and people from dysfunctional families don't believe they have the inherent right to select.

Fourth, *spend time with your partner in two ways:* alone time and in shared social time. You have to build experiences together.

Fifth, *share life experiences*–the more the better. The more history of life experiences you have, the deeper and more intense your relationship is going to be. You do this by doing things together and talking about what that meant to you and how you felt about it. "This is what we did, this is the meaning it had, and this is how I felt about it."

Sixth, *share the breadth of your experiences.* When you do things away from your partner, talk to him or her about your experiences of day-to-day living.

Seventh, *learn how to balance risk-taking and comfort-seeking.* This is critical. Most people who have a tendency toward addictive relationships believe relationships are built on risk-taking—but they aren't. Healthy relationships are built on comfort-seeking, mutual-pleasuring, and satisfaction. Risk-taking occurs in small, measured doses.

Eighth, *learn to talk about two things: what you believe you need and what you want in a relationship.* You need to do reality testing with this, and you can start by talking about it in your ACA group. Once you find a partner, you've got to think, "Here's what I need and here's what I want. I've got to put it into words and be able to tell my partner about it. Then, I have to get interested and concerned about what my partner needs and wants." You must be willing to listen and be concerned about it.

If any partner is unable to know and talk about what they need and want, the process of intimacy collapses. Intimacy is achieving your basic needs so you're comfortable and your basic wants so you're happy.

Ninth, *learn to problem-solve together.* You've got to be willing to involve others in your relationship and ask them for advice. If you're fearful of getting outside help, there's something wrong. In this day and age of changing social norms, morality, and expectations, almost every couple needs a therapist at some time to help sort things out. There is nothing wrong with that. It is, in fact, unhealthy to believe you can maintain an ongoing relationship without ever needing the help of an objective outsider.

Tenth, *make your partner psychologically visible.* Tell him how you see him. Tell her what you think about her, what she means to you, and how you feel about her. Without that, relationships wither and die.

Today's Norm

One monogamous, life-long relationship is no longer typical or perhaps "normal" as it was when the average life expectancy was thirty-six and a man would be married three times between age fourteen and thirty-six because he lost three wives in childbirth. Today, the norm is serial monogamy. In many relationships, we will grow together and outgrow each other, then grow together again and outgrow each other. It's not unusual for people to have three to five primary, substantially enduring relationships in their lives which result in outgrowing each other. There's nothing wrong with that if it's done in a responsible way. You should also recognize that you will attract somebody at your level of growth and that you may grow in unexpected ways.

In summary, know what level of relationship you want and make sure your partner matches that. Evaluate how functional or dysfunctional your relationship is by looking at the eight basic characteristics of addictive relationships and the seven basic counterpoints that occur in healthy relationships. And, finally, know the ways you can begin converting your addictive intimate skills into healthy intimate skills.

Addictive intimacy takes a lot more skill and work than healthy intimacy. If you can engage in an addictive relationship, you can engage in a healthy one. If you believe a relationship has to be an endless series of painful personal-growth experiences, you're never going to have much comfort and satisfaction in your relationships. Once you change that belief by working on yourself and once you learn the basic principles, it will be easier to build healthy intimacy. The intimacy you build will be more satisfying than you ever imagined.